FIT
at
ANY
AGE

Exercise to Stimulate not Annihilate

D0878610

Lee Haney

FIT AT ANY AGE
EXERCISE TO STIMULATE NOT ANNIHILATE

Copyright © 2018 Lee Haney

Published by Book Ripple Publishing
www.BookRipple.com

Photograph acknowledgments:

Jacob Kravtin
kravtinphotography@gmail.com (casual photos)

Afif M. Cherif
Info@studioprimetime.com (exercise photos)

Joshua Bart-Plange
Instagram: @TheClassicLP Website: TheClassicLP.com
Facebook.com/TheClassicLP (recipe photos)

ISBN: 978-1-943157-53-2
Library of Congress Control Number: 2018900766
Printed in the United States of America

To reach the author, go to:
www.LeeHaney.com

WHAT OTHERS ARE SAYING

"I'm happy to endorse my dear friend, Lee Haney's new book. He was Mr. Olympia 8 times and an inductee into the International Sports Hall of Fame. Anyone interested in learning to manage their age through proper exercise and nutrition will benefit greatly from the knowledge Lee shares. He has been there and done it all in the field, and is Icon legend status in the health & fitness industry."

– Dr. Robert M. Goldman MD, PhD, DO, FAASP
World Chairman-International Medical Commission
Co-Founder & Chairman of the Board-A4M
Founder & Chairman-International Sports Hall of Fame
Co-Founder & Chairman-World Academy of Anti-Aging Medicine

"When I was in search of a safe and effective fitness program and trainer, my primary care physician referred me to Mr. Lee Haney. Of course, I knew who Lee Haney was, so I was excited to reach out to him. As expected, he created a program to help meet my fitness goals in a comfortable way. Lee Haney's book offers the perfect plan and guidance for managing age, mobility, and strength the right way."

– Ingrid Saunders Jones
Chairperson
National Council of Negro Women

PREFACE

Forty-plus years of working with people of different ages has given me a clear understanding of what exercise and nutrition should look and feel like for people in their 30's, 40's, 50's, 60's, and older.

Fit at Any Age provides a wealth of knowledge and an online support link to include: workout videos, meal plans, weight loss tips, motivational and inspirational tools to help users reach their fitness goals in a way that safe and effective.

Here's my open invitation to be a part of the greatest Half Time Show ever, by allowing me to serve as your personal Age Management Coach.

– Lee Haney

DEDICATION

This book is dedicated to my second-grade sweetheart and wife, Shirley. She is my WHY for taking care of my health. I can better serve her and my family with a healthy body and a strong mind.

To live long and prosper is the ultimate goal for everyone. However, we must do our part in making that happen. I have everything to live for and to look forward to.

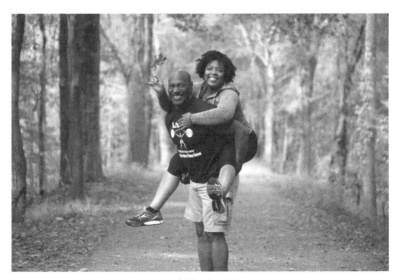

Lee and Shirley Haney

ABOUT THE AUTHOR

As a kid growing up, I would often fantasize about being the biblical judge, Samson, and the mythical legend, Hercules, possessing great strength.

Every physical chore my dad gave me, such as removing rocks from the garden or carrying planks from construction jobs, I welcomed as a way to grow bigger muscles.

At the age of 11, I asked my parents for a set of weights for Christmas. They fulfilled my request with my very own York barbell and dumbbell weight lifting set, which included a Charles Atlas weight lifting brochure.

From that moment on, I read everything I could get my hands on about weight training and nutrition.

Every trip to the grocery or drug store would land me in the magazine section, searching for my favorite body-building stars.

By the time I was 16, I entered my first bodybuilding contest wearing a pair of blue and red underwear from K-Mart. At the time, I didn't know there was such a thing as posing trunks.

My placing in the contest didn't go too well. However, I had fun and was told by the judges I had lots of potential.

The die had been cast for me, a teenager from the small town of Spartanburg, South Carolina, and so began my rise to the top in the field of amateur and professional bodybuilding.

Win History

- 1979 Teen Mr. America – AAU, Overall Winner
- Teen Mr. America – AAU, Tall, 1st
- 1982 Junior Nationals – NPC, Overall Winner
- Junior Nationals – NPC, Heavy Weight, 1st
- Nationals – NPC, Overall Winner
- Nationals – NPC, Heavyweight, 1st
- World Amateur Championships – IFBB, Heavyweight, 1st
- Grand Prix Las Vegas – IFBB, Winner
- Night of Champions – IFBB, Winner
- Olympia – IFBB, Winner
- 1984 Olympia – IFBB, Winner
- 1985 Olympia – IFBB, Winner
- 1986 Olympia – IFBB, Winner
- 1987 Grand Prix Germany IFBB, Winner
- 1988 Olympia – IFBB, Winner
- 1989 Olympia – IFBB, Winner
- 1990 Olympia – IFBB, Winner
- 1991 Olympia – IFBB, Winner

For more info, visit www.leehaney.com

I've often been asked by people, "Was it the training systems, the meal plan, the vitamin supplement program, or the tuna fish that gave you the muscles?"

This is what I believe:

I distinctly recall praying one night before bed, "Lord, if you see fit to make me the best at this sport that I love so much ... I will go before the world and give you the praise and the glory."

Apparently, He heard and answered my prayer in a mighty way. How else can I explain winning the Mr. Olympia title 8 consecutive times and finding a place in the *Guinness Book of World Records*, being appointed as Chairman to the President's Council on Fitness and Sports, being inducted into the International Sports Hall of Fame, hosting exercise shows on both ESPN and the Trinity Broadcast Network (TBN), and the list goes on.

It gives me the greatest pleasure to be able to share the knowledge I gained over the years.

To God be the glory!

– Lee Haney

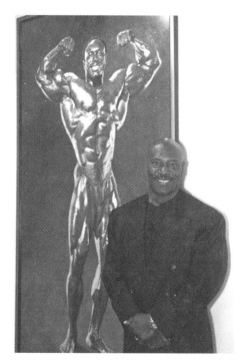

FOREWORD

Having Lee as my personal fitness trainer over the years has made all the difference in my overall health. He is a wealth of knowledge and I strongly recommend his book, *Fit at Any Age.*

You don't get to be an 8-time Mr. Olympia without knowing what you are doing!

– Steve Harvey

CONTENTS

INTRODUCTION

People are now living longer than ever before, as a result of making healthier lifestyle choices. It's common to hear people say, "50 is the new 30," and I, for one, like the way that sounds!

Nothing is going to stop us from aging. From the time we're born, our bodies began to age. And, to our dismay, it never stops. The abs go into hiding, hair starts to thin, eyesight starts to blur, and the joints sounds like a Rice Crispy commercial. "Snap! Crackle! Pop!"

If there were a magic potion for staying young, those of us over 50 would be the first in line to get it. Regrettably, there is no such thing.

On the other hand, there *are* ways to help manage the aging process.

The key to long life and good health is found in quality nutrition, functional exercise, and mental harmony.

If we focus on these three areas of health, being fit at any age is possible. It doesn't matter whether you're 50, or even 90.

My goal is to empower you with the tools to help manage your age

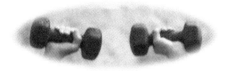

in a way that is simple and easy to apply. Along the way, you will hear some of my most popular training quotes used over the years, to add understanding and clarity while working with a variety of clients. They include:

"Stimulate, not Annihilate" – Exercising to build quality muscle without causing injuries.

"Drive 55 and Stay Alive" – A reminder that you're 55 and not 25. Don't do things that may put you in harm's way while exercising.

"Heat Burn Meat" – It's good to allow your body temperature to rise in order to burn fat better and get rid of stored sodium and impurities.

"Get Your Mind Right" – Put on your I-got-this attitude. Jump in and get the job done. No excuses.

"It's Hard Work Being Cute" – There's a price to pay for feeling good and looking great. If it was easy, everyone would have it.

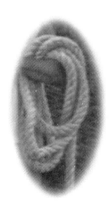

"If you can't Flex It, Don't Carry It" – Watch your weight. If you see yourself putting on extra weight, do something about it.

"In order to Percolate, You Have to Circulate" – Being fit enhances sexual performance. The goal is not just finding ways to age well; it's also about keeping our mojo. Exercise and good nutrition is the best form of Viagra.

"Your Health Is Your Wealth" – There's no greater asset than your health. In order to reap a harvest of good health, we must sow the seeds of good health. We have to be proactive and intentional when it comes to daily exercise and quality nutrition.

"Last Set, Best Set" – Give it your all in everything you set your mind to do, and always find the strength to push through until the task is completed.

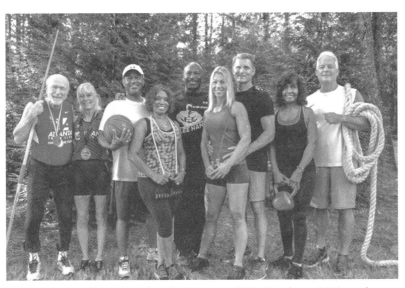

L to R: Bill (90) and wife, Jeanne (80), Paulette (65) and husband, Athaniel (68), Jacklyn (55) and husband, Don (60), Shirley (70), Ken (59), and of course, yours truly (a young and handsome 58, Lee Haney) in the middle. Don't we look good!

Before we get started, I want to call your attention to the picture on the front cover, which features some of my Boomer friends over the age of 50.

They are living proof that it is possible to be fit at any age.

We didn't wake up this morning in this type of shape. It took consistency, and a well-thought-out fitness plan.

You want a plan made up of nutrition, which repairs the body, and exercise, which enhances overall physical function without increasing the risk of injuries.

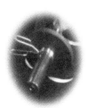

CHAPTER ONE

WHAT OTHERS ARE DOING

All I can say is, "Wow!"

It doesn't get any better than this.

Testimonials and pictures are worth a thousand words. With that being said, what you are about to read should leave you pumped and ready to go!

Enjoy …

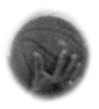

Bill Daprano

When I was a small child, I developed asthma at about the same time my family moved to Austin, Texas. It was during the same period the mid-western part of the United States was suffering the ravages of the great Dust Bowl. This caused Austin to have severe periods of dust storms.

To the asthmatically uninformed, the combination of dust and asthma is like going into an ice locker while suffering from pneumonia. Fortunately, after three years, we moved back to Atlanta. The move from Texas led to an entirely different change in my condition. My new neighborhood had a collection of boys very close to my age. The order of the day was sports from sun up to sun down. During baseball season, it was baseball, and during football season, it was football.

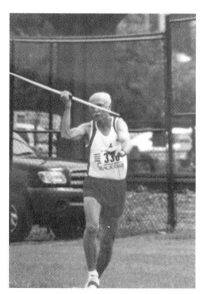

Bill Daprano (90)

My asthma not only got better, it disappeared. Thanks to my new, active lifestyle. It's a lifestyle that I have continued to sustain into my 90s. Without a doubt, I believe staying active and exercising is the most important ingredient to finding the infamous Fountain of Youth. Age management should not only be a choice, but a habit.

Jeanne Daprano

Nutrition and fitness have been such a benefit to this body. I view this body as a living sacrifice, feasting from a diet of whole foods. That means I gradually took things out of my diet that I knew were not living foods. I am still doing this, one thing at a time. I am eating unprocessed foods about 90% of the time. I try not to eat foods that are packaged, so instead, I concentrate on dehydrated foods and living products.

But, without a fitness program, I would not be getting the results in track and field competition I am experiencing. I discipline my body, in order to do physical things that it doesn't want to do. Is it easy? No! But I make it a worship time to my creator, and the commands Jesus gives me.

Here's the bottom line: I try not to put anything into my body or train it in anyway without giving thanks. This means food, drink, and the functional fitness programs are approached with gratitude.

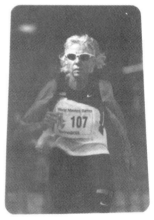

I am not doing this to live longer. With HIS strength, I want to be as effective for the Lord as I can, to honor HIM with how I treat myself this day. I want to be the best I can

Jeanne Daprano (80)

be today, as I run HIS race and finish strong!

Jacklyn Bailey

Health and fitness began at an early age for me; however, I did get off track in my mid 20s when balancing marriage, a full-time career in IT, and having my beautiful daughter. It wasn't until my early 30s that I decided to make a lifestyle change, and think about my health again. I joined a gym and began weight training. I started with a trainer who took me from a moderate size 12 (pear shape) to a size 4 in less than 3 months, by incorporating weight training, cardio, and proper nutrition. I haven't stopped working out since.

To further my zeal for fitness, I begin competing in bodybuilding and figure competitions in my early 40's. The highlight has never been competition. It was the confidence in every area of my life: good health, sound sleep, and endless energy. The icing on the cake is the passion of wellbeing I can pass on to others, by motivating and letting others know it's never too late to make lifestyle changes!

In May 2011, after a 32-year career in IT, I decided it was time to extend my passion for fitness by becoming a Personal Trainer. In July 2011, I received my certification through I.A.F.S. (International Association of Fitness Sciences). I have a strong desire to share this passion of health and fitness with my clients. With compassion and motivation, I hope to help them reach their desired goals.

Here are 10 reasons why I exercise:

1. Self-esteem/confidence
2. Improved health (rare colds or flu)
3. Better sleep – go to sleep quickly!
4. Stronger in daily tasks
5. Energy

6. Healthy skin, hair, and eyes; a more youthful look
7. Weight control
8. Preventive health & longevity
9. Reduces stress/cortisol
10. Flexibility

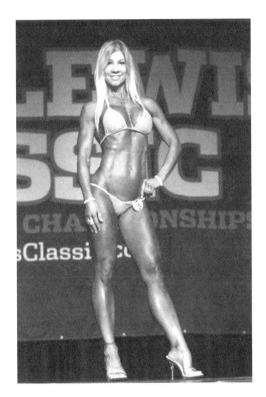

Jacklyn Bailey (55)
NPC Bikini – 2nd – 2014 – 53 yrs
I.A.F.S Certified Personal Trainer
NPC National Physique Competitor

Don Bailey

Exercise and nutrition allow me to do the things I enjoy! At 60, I feel energetic, move well, and sleep well. I'm in the gym a few days a week, but prefer outdoors activities like splitting wood, tinkering on motorcycles, and walking our dog.

About 8 years ago, my wife helped me modify my eating habits. I was eating only 2 meals per day (no breakfast), just a big lunch from the work café and one of those 'healthy' frozen dinners at night. The big lunch left me feeling lethargic in the afternoon.

My wife persuaded me to eat breakfast, and, over time, convinced me to eat between 5 and 6 meals a day.

Now, my body is always fueled, and that gives me the physical and mental clarity to function in all my roles. My workouts emphasize core, and that helps me with the non-gym activities I enjoy.

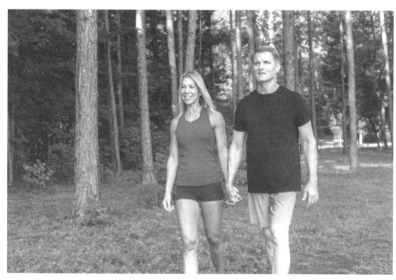

Jacklyn (55) and Don (60) Bailey

Ken Brownlee

Over the past 40 years, exercise and nutrition have greatly benefited me and my lifestyle. I am a muscular build at 6'1", 210 Lbs. I just turned 59 this year, yet I still feel like a 30-year-old.

I have never smoked or drank, I do not take any medications, I am rarely sick, and I have never been admitted to the hospital.

All of my life, I have been fascinated with having muscles and being big and strong. I began buying muscle magazines at age 13 for inspiration, for what would turn out to be my lifelong passion.

At age 15, I started my first workout program. Not too many years after my health journey began, I was fortunate enough to meet and train with the great Lee Haney. To this day, even after all these years, I still follow the same workout routine I began with Lee.

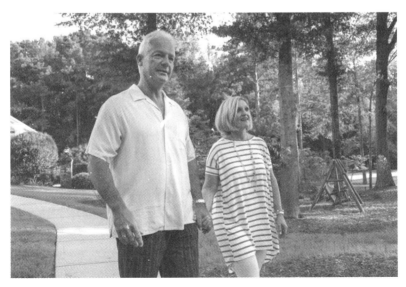

Ken (59) and Lisa (58) Brownlee

At age 50, I began using Lee Haney's Age Management supplements religiously to go along with my diet and exercise routines. The supplements have been a big part of my current overall health, along with years of exercise and healthy eating.

I do not have a specific diet regiment that I follow. I generally try to maintain an overall healthy diet. I never gorge myself. Once I am full, I am done eating. I also follow Lee's advice and try not to over indulge on sweets and fatty foods. The Bible says your body is a temple, and I have always tried to maintain that motto.

Exercise and age management are the true fountains of youth, in my opinion. Maintaining my diet and exercise routines, along with taking Lee Haney's Age Management supplements, has kept my metabolism rate the same.

I may be 59, but aside from the grey hair, I look and feel better than I ever have.

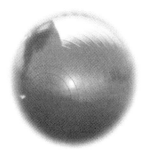

Shirley Johnson

I began working out in my late 40s using the machines, then later incorporated free weights, changed my diet to increase lean protein, and started working out 4 days a week.

When I joined Lee Haney's World Class Fitness Gym, I met Mr. Haney, and he asked me to be a guest on his cable show "Total Lee Fit." Later, he recommended me for a segment that Fox 5 news was doing: "Women Working Out with Weights."

I continue to work out 4 days a week. My weekly routine consists of lifting free weights, some machines, jumping rope, hitting the speed bag, pull ups, bench press, dumb bell press, push-ups, leg press, and leg extensions.

I have learned it takes a combination of commitment, a daily work out regiment, and a smart diet plan to achieve my goal, which is a lifestyle of good health and maximum results.

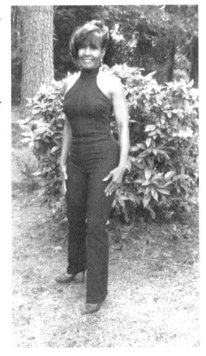

Shirley Johnson (70)

Paulette King

Exercise and nutrition have been a vital part of my life for many years. I love to work out! As a child, I was introduced to gymnastics and swimming, which helped to whet my appetite for exercise.

As a result of staying in shape and maintaining a healthy diet, at the age of 65, I am not on any medication. No high blood pressure, no diabetes, no heart disease, and no other health issues that typically pounce on you as a senior. I am very energetic, and I feel like a 30-year-old, youthful in my appearance and thought life.

As a woman, a stylish wardrobe can be easily maintained when you're in shape. My husband and I share the same love of exercise, which is awesome for our marriage!

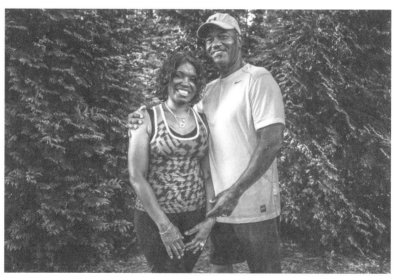

Paulette (65) and Athaniel (68) King

Athaniel King

I have been into exercise since the age of 15. I played football in high school, and followed that with a 33-year military career. Exercise has always been a way of life for me. I enjoy being physically fit, so when I retired from the military and my civilian job, I continued to work out 4 to 5 times a week.

Once I discovered soda and beer are not good sources to replenish the fluids lost during a long run or a lengthy tennis match, I turned to water as my main source of hydration. If I have one weakness when it comes to a balanced diet, it's an occasional chocolate cookie.

My wife prepares our meals to be low sodium, low starch, and we have no fried foods. So, my eating habits have improved during our marriage. Exercise and eating a balanced diet have allowed me to feel good and continue to do things I've enjoyed for most of my 68 years. I recently attended my 50th class reunion, and I adore all of those who were in attendance. I must say, it felt good to show off my 32" waistline. I'm not bragging; I'm just saying if you work out, it shows.

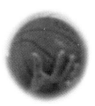

CHAPTER TWO

WHAT ABOUT YOU?

When it comes to exercise and nutrition, I've seen it all. I have also worked with world-class athletes like Evander Holyfield, NFL Super Bowl winner Shannon Sharpe, TV talk show personality Steve Harvey, world-class Master's Track and Field athletes Bill (90 yrs.) and Jeanne Daprano (80 yrs.), and super mom Renee Casey (53 yrs.), who is a wife, mom, grandmother, veteran, and cancer survivor.

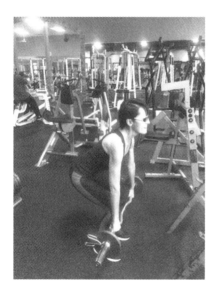

Renee Casey (53)

I guess you could say, "I've been there, done that." Not to say I know everything. However, I do have quite an impressive resume, to say the least.

The philosophy needed to learn the correct way in putting together an exercise and nutrition program is not rocket science.

However, in today's information-driven society, it's easy to get confused and become overwhelmed.

That's okay. Help is on the way.

I will help you establish a lifestyle exercise and fitness program that can last you a lifetime. One that will give you the tools needed to manage your age, and get the greatest of quality and quantity during your life.

Before we get started, let's get your mind right!

In order to be successful doing anything, you have to have a made-up mind, and the right information.

There must always be a purpose behind everything you do, and a strong "Why" behind it. With your end goal in mind, find your own personal "Why," for taking care of your health.

For me, my "Why" is about feeling good and staying pretty. Since taking personal ownership of my health, I have yet to complain of being sick with colds, viruses, or other common health ailments.

I'm conscious of the fact that good health directly impacts my ability to gain wealth. Those of us that work for a living or run our own companies realize the security of our families and businesses depend upon us staying healthy. Good health and wealth co-exist, just as poor health and poverty does.

Indeed, your health is your wealth!

My other "Why" has to do with staying alive to take care of my family.

Make a determination of your own personal "Why." Once you've locked it in, you're ready to go. Own it!

The goal of every fitness program should be to "Stimulate, not annihilate!"

Try to forget some of the crazy exercise rhetoric passed down over the years. One being, "No Pain, No Gain!" That wasn't meant for the average person. It was created by, and for, insane people like me. When I entered the weight room, I wanted to terrorize my opponents. I wanted to make them feel inferior, and to think, "I could never beat the great Lee Haney, he's too awesome."

The proper way to engage health and fitness should be implemented in a lifestyle approach.

Too often, people get involved in exercises and diet programs that are more than their mind and body can tolerate.

For example, let's look at Mrs. Smith. She's a 35-year-old at 5'2" and 175 pounds, wanting to get involved in training for the first time. Her goal is to lose weight, feel better about how she looks, and have more energy. She has only 30 minutes to train each day.

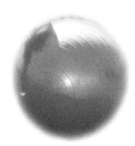

Her program should be in line with her present condition, not consist of exercises that are high-impact and over bearing, such as jumping ropes, running stadium steps, running, walking lunges, box jumps, and plyometrics, to name a few.

Being 5'2" and 175 pounds presents a challenge. Carrying more weight than her frame is meant to carry is her first concern.

According to the American Arthritis Organization, for every pound you weigh over your recommended weight scale, 4 lbs. of additional weight is being placed on your lower body.

For instance, if you're carrying 40 lbs. more than you should, you've added 160 lbs. (40x4) of additional weight on your joints. This can result in joint pain in the knees, hips, or lower back.

Mrs. Smith needs a fitness plan that suits her every-day lifestyle. One that incorporates strength exercises, to help her develop lean muscle.

Muscle is important in keeping her skeletal system strong, and helping her body burn calories more efficiently.

She will also benefit by using a series of core exercises to keep her core strong. These are the muscles found in the abdominal and lower back areas. They will help her maintain good balance as she ages.

She'll also need exercises to enhance her cardio condition. There's a saying: "It's better to have, and not need, than to need, and not have."

There is also the importance of maintaining a certain level of flexibility. People are constantly getting injured by something as small as reaching for an item.

This is why Mrs. Smith's lifestyle program must include stretching.

Each of the exercises mentioned can be set up to give Mrs. Smith exactly what she needs, without causing her extreme discomfort, or the need to have a degree in exercise science.

The same exercise philosophy for Mrs. Smith works for the guys as well.

The goal is still the same: "Stimulate, not Annihilate!" It's all about lifestyle and managing age.

Guys have to work on keeping our ego in check. As men, we're always in a contest to determine who will be the Alpha Male.

We all desire to be that guy, the one who lifts the heaviest weights and sports the coolest set of biceps. After all, the ladies love 'em.

There's nothing wrong with a healthy ego. It's a great motivational tool.

However, the ego must be tempered with wisdom. "You got to know when to hold them, and when to fold them." (Great wisdom from the Gambler!)

Now that we have a good grasp concerning the correct philosophy for exercise, let's discuss nutrition.

CHAPTER THREE

NUTRITION AT ANY AGE

When it comes to nutrition, we need to be sure we have a clear understanding of what's needed to repair our bodies and supply energy. We need to know what to eat, when to eat, how much to eat, and how to put it all together.

Nutrition accounts for 75% of being able to reach your fitness goals. If quality nutrition isn't present in the body, it's nearly impossible to function on any level.

Our focus should be on the foods that nourish the body and help to remove waste in the process. I like to refer to them as "in and out foods." These are foods that do their job, and do not linger in our system, creating waste and bloat.

We're all familiar with the saying, "You are what you eat." If your everyday existence consists of a diet filled with garbage food, there's a strong chance that your time here on earth will not be long.

The body is the most amazing machine ever created. It has the ability to heal itself. After a good night of sleep, it reboots for another day of physical and mental activities. Plus, it has this incredible, God-given ability to manufacture people.

The following information will help you establish a good foundation concerning the function of protein, carbo-hydrates, and fats. In turn, this will also give you a better understanding of the purpose of each of them, and the roles they play in keeping us healthy. We will also learn about the benefits of various herbs and other nutrients, and the importance of quality water— "Nature's Nectar."

Protein:

> Protein is key to building and maintaining quality muscle tissue. Muscle is important for strength-ening our skeletal system, and helps the body burn calories more efficiently. Known as the building blocks for the body, protein is absolutely necessary in repairing cells and tissue.

There are several forms of protein that can be used when putting together a good nutritional program. It may consist of chicken, fish, beef, dairy, vegetable sources, and protein supplements. With a variety of these protein sources in our diet, we will have what is needed for a strong and healthy body.

The following are my top protein recommendations:

- Salmon (i.e. wild Alaskan—high in omega oil)

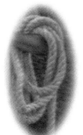

- Sea Bass (high in omega oil)
- Mackerel (high in omega oil)
- Halibut, Cod, Grouper, Flounder, Snapper, Trout
- Chicken (raised without hormones or antibiotics)
- Cottage cheese (low sodium)

- Eggs (raised on natural vegetable sources, without hormones or antibiotics)
- Beans: (i.e. Crowder peas, field peas, navy beans, red beans, pinto beans, black beans, butter beans—great sources of protein that include carbohydrates for energy, and fiber for fighting cholesterol)

Fish was at the top of the list because it's one of the few protein sources that hasn't been tainted with hormones and antibiotics. Besides, I like the nutritional examples Jesus used in making fish His number one protein source when eating with His disciples. Apparently, He knew something about quality nutrition!

Red meat isn't one of my favorites because of the amount of time it takes to digest; however, having it once a week isn't the end of the world. Remember, we want food sources that are in and out, and not those that linger.

How much protein should you consume per serving?
I recommend no more than 20-30 grams per serving for the average person. Since we're concerned with age management and not training for "Mr. Olympia," 40-75 total grams per day is all that's needed. For ladies, I recommend 40-45 grams per day. For men, 50-75 grams. Keep in mind the main function of protein is to build muscle and repair cells.

In some cases, I recommend leaning toward plant-based proteins, such as beans, lentils, and quinoa. They contain fiber, which is important in ridding the body of waste. This is especially true for those who are dealing with slow bowel movements.

Carbohydrates: *Carbohydrates* are important when it comes to fueling the body with energy. They are also a key component when it comes to weight loss. The amount of carbohydrates needed for daily caloric intake varies depending upon individual activity level.

For instance, someone that has a physically demanding job will need more carbohydrates than someone who doesn't. When I trained for competition, I would consume 300-500 grams of carbohydrates a day. Now that I'm over age 50 and spend a lot more time at my desk, I consume less than half of that amount. In short, for those of us who do not work like UPS delivery drivers, keep the carbohydrate intake low!

For the average adult male, I recommend 100-150 grams of carbohydrates per day. For the average female, I recommend 50-75 grams per day. These amounts, respectively, will give us the energy we need, and will not leave a surplus hanging out in our bodies to be converted to fat.

A good indication to know what your body may need is found in your energy level during the day. If you lack energy, it's possible your carbohydrate intake could be too low. In that case, add, for example, fruit—such as an apple or a pear. However, you must also take into account how much sleep you're getting. I recommend getting at 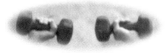 least 6-7 hours per night. Sleep is important, because it helps the body repair itself.

On the other hand, toxins and waste can rob you of energy. If stored waste or toxins are the problem, a seven-day systemic cleansing and detox program can be used to re-energize the body. Either could cause energy loss, which will further increase the craving for more carbohydrates.

Keep in mind that, the fewer carbohydrates needed to power your day, the easier it is to burn body fat and control your weight. Another key thing to remember is to not deprive your body of carbohydrates, since they are your number one source of healthy energy at any age.

There are two categories of carbohydrates: complex carbs and simple carbs. Complex carbs are the ones we should concern ourselves with the most. They consist of foods like pasta, brown rice, grains, corn, and sweet potatoes. When the goal is either weight loss or weight maintenance, we must limit these types of carbohydrates.

The better choice of carbohydrates for those who want to control or lose weight is found in fruit. It tastes great and burns fast, while offering fiber that helps fight cholesterol. Here's my top list of fruits:

- Pears (unpeeled—loaded with fiber)
- Apples (unpeeled)
- Pineapple (excellent source of fiber/supplement for digestive enzymes)
- Papaya (excellent source of fiber/supplement for digestive enzymes)
- Strawberries (antioxidants)

- Blueberries and Blackberries (the perfect antioxidants for cellular health)
- Oranges (great source of vitamin C to boost immune system)
- Watermelon and Cantaloupe (great low-calorie snacks)

While this is a recommended list of good-tasting carbohydrates, be sure to incorporate those best suited for your taste buds. But remember, these are still carbohydrates, and they can be converted to fat if they are not utilized to power our activities.

There are also high fiber/low-calorie leafy carbohydrates that make a world of difference in our total physical well-being. If it were not for these bountiful treasures, toxins would reap havoc throughout our entire body!

I can clearly recall, as a youngster, sopping up the last bit of collard green juice with cornbread left over from the meals my mother would prepare. Greens are the perfect food for flushing waste out of the body, besides castor oil. And today, they still serve the same purpose!

Below is a recommended list of awesome veggies that will help keep our bodies healthy while fighting off toxins:

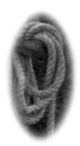

- Collard greens
- Cabbage
- Turnip greens
- Squash
- Spinach
- Kale
- Celery

- Broccoli
- Green beans
- Green peas
- Okra
- Lettuce
- Tomatoes
- Asparagus
- Cauliflower
- Chard

Another form of carbohydrates we must be cautious of are high-calorie, caffeinated energy beverages, which can cause weight gain and raise blood pressure. There's a ton of them on the market. Having energy should be a result of proper rest and quality nutrition, not synthetic substances. When needing an extra push or wake me up, I rely on a cup of coffee or hot tea with lemon and honey.

Fats:
Fats play an important role in our overall health, just as protein and carbohydrates. There are basically two types of fats we should be aware of: saturated and unsaturated. Saturated fats come from animal sources, which can raise bad cholesterol levels. Unsaturated fats come from plant sources, which are known to fight bad cholesterol. Another beneficial source of fat is found in fish oil—also known as omega-3. Fish oil has been used to reduce blood pressure, fight arthritis, and lower cholesterol.

When choosing the best sources of fat for my diet, I prefer to use the combination of nuts and oils high in essential fatty acids.

Here are my top choices:

Walnuts:
>Walnuts are at the top of my list, because they are easy to find, and add texture to my oatmeal. They also offer support for increased cardiovascular health.

Brazil nuts:
>Brazil nuts are an excellent in-between meals snack, and are high in the mineral selenium, which is used to help fight cancer. I consume 5-10 Brazil nuts a day.

Almonds:
>Almonds are the most widely used nuts in the world. Not only are they easy to find, they are great for fighting hunger pains, and are low in saturated fat. They are an excellent source of vitamin E, calcium, magnesium, and iron. Health experts also recommend almonds for fighting heart disease and cancer.

There are other nut choices that also offer good health benefits; however, the three discussed above are my favorites! As for omega oils that can be used to prepare or compliment food, canola, safflower, and coconut oils are the most popular. All three are used to help fight bad cholesterol.

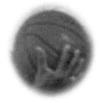

When I want a quick, nutritious meal, I choose one out of the three for stir frying.

Olive oil:

Olive oil is in a class of its own when it comes to giving the body the best of friendly, cholesterol-fighting omegas.

Now, let's put it all together to create some delicious meals from recipes that are easy to prepare and digest.

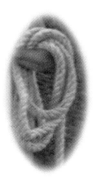

Baked Fresh Herb Salmon with Grilled Asparagus and Brown Rice

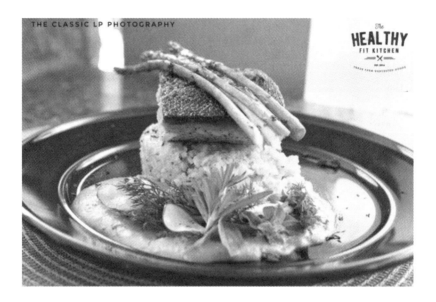

- 6-oz. salmon
- 14 asparagus spears
- 1 cup (8 oz.) steamed brown rice
- Fresh tarragon
- Fresh basil
- Fresh Rosemary
- 2 oz. olive oil

Instructions:

Step 1: Pre-heat oven to 350 degrees, bundle all herbs together, and mince herbs with a knife until all is one.

Step 2: Rub herb medley all over the salmon with olive oil.

Step 3: Oil sauté skillet with olive oil (1 ounce).

Allow oil to get hot, then place salmon in cooking skillet skin side down, and cover for 6-7 minutes. Uncover and turn salmon over, skin side up. Then, use tongs and remove. Peel skin completely off and place to the side. Now, recover salmon with top and allow to sear for 3-4 minutes.

Step 4: Remove from the skillet and allow salmon to finish cooking in the oven for 7-8 minutes.

Step 5: Rinse off asparagus, then drizzle or spray with olive oil. When grill is hot, lay spears on the grill until slightly charred, and remove.

Step 6: Rinse and drain brown rice. Place in rice cooker. Cover with a cup of water and let it cook 15-20 minutes, until tender and fluffy.

Ready to eat!

Baked Cod with Quinoa and Kale

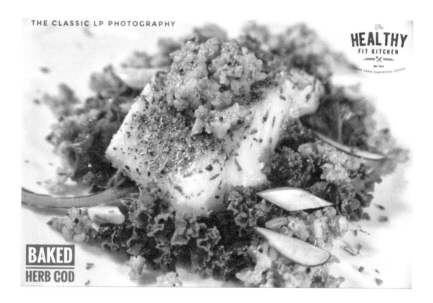

- 8oz Cod
- 1 cup spiced quinoa
- 2 cups of kale
- 1 ounce of oregano
- 1 ounce of basil
- 1 ounce of minced garlic
- 2 tbsp. of olive oil
- 1 tbsp. sea salt
- 1 tbsp. of pepper

Instructions:

Step 1: Preheat oven to 350 degrees. Add 1tbsp. olive oil in cooking pan and allow to get hot, until it slightly boils.

Step 2: Season both sides of cod fish with oregano, basil, garlic, and salt & pepper. Place down in cooking pan and allow both sides to sear slightly. Finish off in the oven for 10-15 minutes.

Step 3: Boil water and add a teaspoon of olive oil and a pinch of sea salt. Once the water comes to a boil, add in the quinoa, the garlic, basil, and oregano. Stir slowly and allow it to boil for 20-25 minutes, until quinoa is fluffy. Add salt and pepper to taste and stir. Ready to plate.

Step 4: Rinse kale in cold water bath. Place in steamer for 3-4 minutes. Don't allow kale to lose its color and its crunch.

Ready to eat!

Blackened Grilled Ahi Tuna with Roasted Zucchini, Asparagus, and Baked Sweet Potato

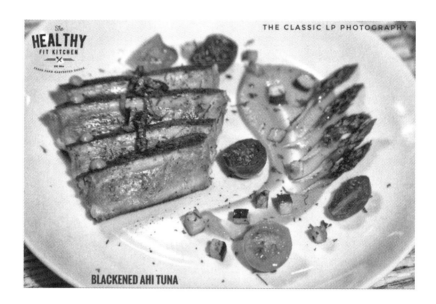

- 6 oz. Ahi Tuna
- 1 cup Fresh Zucchini
- 6 Asparagus Spears
- 1/2 Cup Sweet Potatoes
- 1 tsp of Basil
- 1 tsp of Oregano
- 1 tsp of Paprika
- 1 tsp of Garlic
- 1 tsp of Pepper Corns
- 1 tsp olive oil

Instructions:

Step 1: Season both sides of the 6 oz. Ahi Tuna so it's completely covered on both sides.

Step 2: Pour olive oil into a cooking pan and heat

at a medium temperature until hot.

Step 3: Place seasoned tuna into skillet until seared on both sides for 3-4 minutes on each side until a blackened crust has formed. Remove tuna from pan. It should have a pink middle, as if it was medium temperature cooked. Place to the side and wrap while waiting to plate.

Step 4: Angle chop the zucchini into slices and rinse with water.

Step 5: Cut only the green parts of the asparagus and be sure to disregard the bottom of the spear that is white.

Step 6: Medley all the cut asparagus, along with the zucchini. Season with sea salt, black pepper, and oregano.

Step 7: Place in oven at 350 degrees for 20-25 minutes to add a roasted flavor to the veggies. When removed, allow them to cool.

Step 8: Clean and cut the potato the long way, place on a cooking sheet, and place in oven at 400 degrees. Baking the sweet potato will take at least 40 minutes. To speed up the process, you can boil the potato to produce a softer texture, then bake it faster. Add cinnamon and nutmeg for flavoring and garnish.

Ready to eat!

Oven Baked Sirloin Steak with Sweet Potato and Green Beans

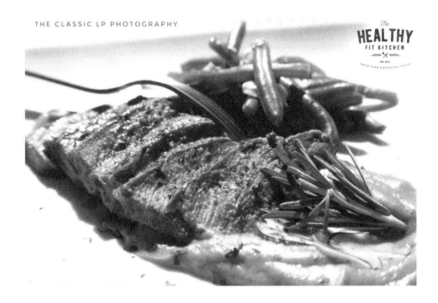

- 6-8oz sirloin cut steak
- 3-4oz Boiled Sweet Potato
- 1.5 cup steamed green beans
- 1 tsp of paprika
- 1 tsp of cumin
- 1 tsp of sea salt
- 1 tsp black pepper
- 1 tbsp. olive oil

Instructions:

Step 1: Pre-heat oven to 350 degrees. Begin to mix all seasonings in a bowl until they all are incorporated as one.

Step 2: Apply rub to both sides of the sirloin. In cooking pan, heat olive oil until it slightly bubbles, then apply steak to cooking pan. Sear for 2 minutes on both sides. Remove and place in baking tray and finish cooking in the oven for another 15 minutes, until it is medium well.

Step 3: Rinse and boil sweet potato for 40 minutes. Remove from water and peel off the skin. Place in mixing bowl and mash.

Step 4: Rinse green beans and place in boiling water no more than 8-10 minutes. Remove from hot water and insert into an ice bowl with cold water (shocking to stop cooking). Leave in water for 6-8 minutes then remove and sprinkle a pinch of sea salt.

Ready to eat!

Sweet & Spicy Chicken Stir Fry

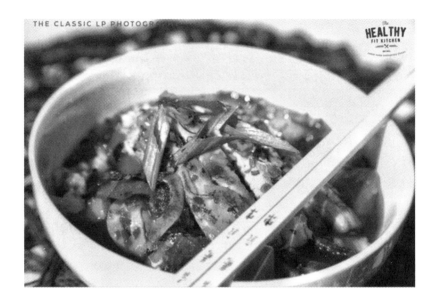

- 4 oz. Chicken Breast
- 1/2 of a Red Onion
- 1 Red Bell Pepper
- 1 Green Bell Pepper
- 1/4 cup of sliced green onions
- 1/2 cup liquid aminos
- 1 tsp. Sesame Oil
- 1 tbsp. Rice Vinegar
- 1 tbsp. Sweet Chili Sauce
- 1 cup of Brown Rice

Instructions:

Step 1: Slice chicken breast into chopped slivers.

Step 2: Place into cooking pan, add sea salt and pepper, and cook until done. Cook time 8-10 minutes. Place to the side when done.

Step 3: Cut onions, both peppers, and green onions into long slivers.

Step 4: In a cooking pot or wok, combine liquid aminos, sesame oil, rice vinegar, and sweet chili sauce.

Step 5: Heat up all liquids at a high temperature, until liquids began to simmer. Allow liquids to heat up for 6-7 minutes, then reduce heat.

Step 6: Place all other ingredients, as well as your cooked chicken breast, and allow to cook for 10-12 minutes.

Step 7: Boil water. Add in teaspoon of sea salt, stir, then add rice to boiling water. Cook until water is reduced and rice is tender and fluffy.

Step 8: Plate rice first, then add meat and veggies over the rice, then pour over broth.

Ready to eat!

Easy Made Pulled Chicken Stir Fry

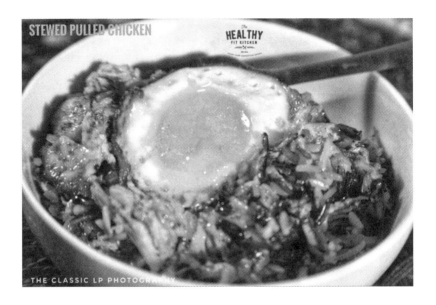

- 1 cup cooked rice
- 2 tbsp. of soy sauce
- 1 tsp. of Grade-A Honey
- 1 tsp of ground ginger
- 1 garlic clove
- 1 tsp of red pepper flakes
- 4 oz. chicken breast (sliced)
- 1 tbsp. olive oil
- 1 cup Broccoli crowns
- 1/2 cup sliced carrots
- 1/2 medium onion (diced)
- 1 whole egg

Instructions: Chicken Breast
> **Step 1:** Pre-heat oven to 375-380 degrees. Place chicken breast on baking pan. Season with sea salt and black pepper.

Step 2: Pour 1 tablespoon olive oil over the breast and cover with aluminum foil. Place in oven and bake for 30 minutes.

Step 3: When done, pull from oven and uncover. Grab two forks and begin to shred chicken breast into thin slices until completely shredded.

Step 4: In a sauté skillet or large cooking pan, place all ingredients (except chicken) and cook vegetables at a medium temperature.

Step 5: Next, add chicken and mix until all has come together as a stir fry. This will cook for up to 10-15 minutes.

Step 6: Pour over steamed rice, preferably basmati rice.

Instructions: Fried Egg

Step 1: Place a teaspoon of olive oil in frying pan.

Step 2: Allow pan to get very hot at medium setting, then crack and add egg

Step 3: Egg should be done in about 3-4 minutes. Only fry on one side. Egg white edges should begin to brown.

Step 4: Remove with spatula and place on top of the stir fry dish.

Ready to eat!

There you have it!

These meals not only taste good, they are good for you!

Our compliments and special thanks to Chef Yasin! Here is his contact information:

www.chefyasinkcorder.com
www.thehealthyfitkitchen.com
Instagram.com/chefyasinkcorder
Instagram.com/thehealthyfitkitchen.com
Facebook - Yasin.Corder

CHAPTER FOUR

AGE MANAGEMENT SUPPLEMENTATION

Now more than ever, vitamins and herbs are being used for physical well-being. With the high cost of medical insurance and prescription medicine, people are looking for other alternatives. It doesn't matter whether you're a homemaker, business professional, or an athlete, supplementation is beneficial and necessary. After all, they existed long before institutionalized medicine.

A well-rounded nutritional program should begin with a natural food base, multi-vitamin, and multi-mineral combination. Vitamins are essential in giving the body important nutrients that we may lack in our daily nutritional intake. Nutrients help repair cells, muscle function, aid in digestion, restore energy, aid in mental clarity, strengthen bones, and boost the immune system.

The following is a list of nutrients that offer health benefits to help manage age:

Trans-resveratrol:
Used to fight heart disease

D-3:
Used to increase bone health, brain clarity, and balance insulin

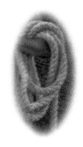

Ubiquinol:
Used to increase stamina and recovery

Omega fish oil:
Used for cardio-vascular health

Joint complex (MSM, Glucosamine, Chondroitin, Shark Cartilage):
Used for joint health

All of the age management nutrients mentioned are present in my "Age Management Pack," which can be found at www.leehaney.com.

I also highly recommend probiotics, a great form of supplementation. Probiotics consist of a complex of cultured friendly bacteria that aid in digestion and boost the immune system. Let's just say, it's great stuff!

Herbal supplements:
Herbs have been around since the beginning of time. They were man's first medicines. There are herbs for nearly every type of sickness or disease; however, the biggest use is for disease prevention. It would be nearly impossible to name all the different herbs and how they're to be used, especially when many of them have several medicinal purposes.

My top herbal remedies are Echinacea and Golden Seal,

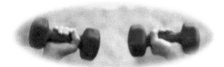 used to help boost the immune system when it's being attacked.

A great source of herbal information is available in the book *Prescription for Nutritional Healing* by Phyllis A. Balch, CNC. It has been a tremendous resource to me over the years. Having knowledge of herbs and how they are used can have a positive impact on our present and long-term health.

Some of the most frequently used herbs are found in my 7-Day Systemic Cleansing and Detox program. Detoxification has proven to be a great way to keep the body energized and refreshed. It helps get rid of stored waste and bloat, which leaves the body tired and sluggish. It also aids in the health of the internal organs, such as the kidney, liver, urinary system, cleansing of the blood stream, and the colon.

Detoxing the body is similar to having our cars serviced every 3,500 miles. By keeping the oil and filter clean, we stand a greater chance of getting better gas mileage, and the engine lasting longer. The body is no different.

The following is a list of herbs that are part of my 7-day systemic cleansing and detox program offered by "Lee Haney's Nutritional Support System," which can be found at www.leehaney.com.

Herbal cleansing complex for the Blood, Liver, Kidney, Urinary system

- Milk Thistle (blood cleanser)
- Burdock Root
- Yellow Dock
- Red Clover

- Golden Seal
- Cranberry Powder extract
- Garlic
- Lemon extract

Colon cleansing fiber complex

- Oat Bran
- Bentonite Clay
- Glucomannan
- African Bird Pepper
- Fennel Seed
- Senna Leaves
- Cape Aloe
- Cascara Sagrada
- Flax Seed oil

Systemic cleansing and detoxing has proven to be an excellent health tool for ridding the body of waste and toxins.

How often should someone detox their body?
At least twice a year; however, if you're in a constant struggle with junk food, red meat, and processed food, every quarter is recommended.

For the past decade, Lee Haney's Nutritional Support System has promoted what is known as "The 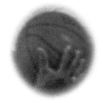 Transformation Now Challenge," to help people struggling with weight issues get back on track. The many testimonials have been nothing short of incredible. Visit www.leehaney.com for testimonials.

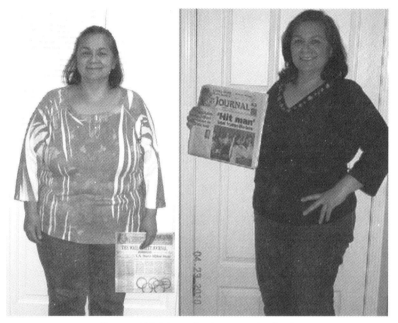

Susan Webber (before and after)

Check out this before and after photo! Susan was one of our recent Transformation winners. She lost over 25 pounds in 30 days. Anything is possible when you get your mind right.

Water:
> This is the most valuable natural resource known to man. Without it, we cannot exist. The body weight of an adult is made up of 75% water. Water has several functions in the body. It's important for digestion, it keeps the body temperature under control, it flushes waste products through the system, transports nutrition, and helps the body maintain proper lubrication, to name a few benefits.

It's recommended that we drink at least eight 8 oz. glasses of water per day to remain hydrated. For someone who's involved in a lot of physical activity or working in the sun, more is needed. The best indication is your thirst. At every opportunity during the day, we should make a conscious effort to drink water.

It is best to drink water at either cool or room temperature. We've all experienced brain freeze at some point. It's not a good feeling, and can be harmful.

What is the best form of water?
Well, the jury is still deliberating that question.

Out in the country where I grew up, we relied on well and spring water. These days I don't advise well water that hasn't been tested for safety. The better choices are alkaline, spring, or purified water. My first choice is certified spring water. It's the perfect medicine, so drink up and enjoy!

10 Nutritional Tips

The following are 10 nutritional tips proven to be beneficial:

1. Eat for what you are going to be doing, not for what you have done. This means the majority of your calories should be taken in during the active part of your day. Most of us are active between 8:00 a.m. - 4:00 p.m.

2. Be cautious of foods high in fat and complex carbohydrates, such as French fries, pizza, pasta, potatoes, breads, etc., when your goal is to lose body fat or drop a few pounds.

3. Stay away from zero carbohydrate diets. These types of diets can cause memory lapse, slow bowel movement, fatigue, the loss of muscle, and light-headedness.

4. Do not skip meals when trying to lose weight. This throws the metabolic clock off balance. As children, our bodies were programmed for three main meals per day (breakfast, lunch, and dinner). When that sequence is not followed, the body throws up its own defense mechanism by holding on to fat, in order to protect itself.

5. If you can't flex it, don't carry it. Keep a tab on the scale and mirror. If the body fat starts to increase, cut back, and stop avoiding mirrors. Excess body weight can cause joint problems as we age. Let the last meal of the evening be fruit or a mixed salad with low calorie dressing. Don't forget the water!

6. Keep a nutritional calorie journal. By measuring your calorie intake, you will know whether to add or take away. This is key when wanting to drop some unwanted pounds.

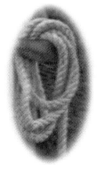

7. Compare labels for nutritional information on products when

grocery shopping. Be especially aware of the fat, carbohydrate, and sodium content.

8. Eat four to five small meals a day instead of three large meals. The body will burn the calories more efficiently, and the craving for food will not be as great. Keep in mind a meal can be the size of a banana, apple, bran muffin, or a cup of yogurt.

9. Never wait until you're starving before having a meal. You are most likely to overeat during that time. Always have a healthy snack between meals, such as an apple, pear, banana or a few nuts (i.e., walnuts, almonds, brazil nuts).

10. Break the age-old habit of eating everything on your plate. When the portions are large, leave with a slight feeling of satisfaction verses being full!

Remember, it is important to feed your body quality nutrition. Proper nutrition accounts for 75% of who we are, and our goal is to remember "you are what you eat." The body is on a never-ending quest to generate new cells and tissue. That process is cut short when empty and worthless calories are given to the body.

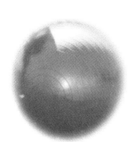

When quality food is put into the body, quality performance will be the result! You can only get out what you put in.

CHAPTER FIVE

GETTING RID OF EXCESS WEIGHT

There is a difference between healthy and unhealthy weight. Lean muscle weight is important in keeping your skeletal system strong, and helping the body burn calories efficiently.

However, a high percentage of body fat can convert to estrogen, which can create series of health issues such as cancer, diabetes, heart disease, U.F. (Uterus Fibroids) and E.D. (Erectile Dysfunction), to name a few.

The key to getting rid of unwanted weight and body fat is not allowing it to sneak up on you. Start with small steps, like getting rid of sugary drinks and snacks. A glass of sweet tea can have as many as 300 calories. A bag of chips as many as 275 calories. This alone can help you drop one pound a week.

Take time to plan your meals. Most people make bad choices when they're eating on the go.

Make it a priority to keep healthy, low-calorie food and snacks around the house, work, and in the car. That way, you're not setting yourself up for failure.

Don't take in more calories than you're going to burn. Especially when it comes to carbohydrates. Carbs are energy foods. They are there to strengthen you for the physical demands of your daily activities.

For many of us, the daily activities never happen. The body then stores the carbs. Over a period of time, the unused calories convert to fat. When your activities are low, so should your carb intake be.

Try to stay away from self-inflected temptations, like having snacks around the house, or hanging out with friends who always want to eat out. Try the opposite approach by suggesting a trail walk through the park, or an evening of bowling.

When exercising, do your best to get some direct sunlight when it's early and cool outside. Your body will appreciate the vitamin D-3. It's also important that the body develops a bearable tolerance for heat. A good sweat is the perfect medicine for getting rid of toxins and sodium. Heat also raises the metabolism, to help burn calories.

When training clients, I often shout, "Heat Burns Meat!"

As an example, I have them imagine a slab of ribs being cooked on the grill. As the heat rises, the fat slowly melts 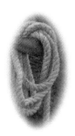 away. This is the same principle behind a well-organized, functional training workout, incorporating strength, core, stretching, and cardio in the same set, to raise the body temperature to help burn fat.

Embrace the heat! But, be careful. Don't have a stroke. Remember, "Stimulate, not annihilate!"

Don't buy into the excuse it's your thyroid that's causing you to gain weight. Ask yourself if you've ever recalled seeing an obese person, in a third world country, with a thyroid problem?

Right! Not a one. A body will not and cannot grow without nutrition. Bad or good. In short, "If you don't put it in, you won't have to take it off."

Below is a meal plan I created for people wanting to make healthy lifestyle changes. It's simple and straight to the point. This particular meal plan was created with the same eating principles in mind, given with my 10 nutritional tips.

With the information you've acquired, you are now empowered to make changes where needed. Yes, you have homework. If the amount of food recommended leaves you a bit bloated, cut back. Nothing is etched in stone. Listen to your body.

Choice Meal Plan

Breakfast: Choice #1
1-2 whole eggs (boiled or scrambled w/coconut oil) flavored w/ pepper
Half of a medium apple or pear w/skin
Glass of water w/lemon (fresh squeezed wedges)

Breakfast: Choice #2

Omelets (1 whole egg and 3 whites) may include: onions, mushrooms, peppers, tomatoes) cooked w/a small amount of olive oil or safflower oil
Low sodium salsa can be added for flavor if needed.
Small cup of mixed berries
Glass of water w/lemon

Snack:

3 Brazil nuts or 4-6 walnut halves
Glass of water w/lemon

Lunch: Choice #1

Sautéed Chicken 4oz. or a broiled turkey patty
Medium mixed salad (lettuce or mixed greens, tomatoes, cucumber, carrots, mushroom, onions, apple or pear wedges 3-4)
Dressing preferred is vinaigrette
Glass of water w/lemon

Lunch: Choice #2

Plant base protein shake (1 scoop w/ 30 calorie Almond milk)

Snack: Choice #1

Small cup of blue berries or straw berries
Glass of water w/lemon

Snack: Choice #2

Medium apple
Glass of water w/ lemon

Dinner: Choice #1

White fish (baked, grilled, or broiled) 3-4oz.
Mixed sautéed veggies (squash, zucchini, onions, peppers, tomatoes, carrots)
Veggies can be flavored or prepared with smoked turkey, pepper, Mrs. Dash, and safflower oil.

* Try to avoid using salt. Sea salt if you must.
* Dinner meal should be consumed by 7:30 or 8pm.
* If you get the munchies, have a mixed green salad, same as the lunch selection.

These meals keep the carbohydrates low, to force the body to burn fat. I also kept the fiber high, to eliminate waste. The success rate has been extremely high using this particular plan.

There is room to make substitutes to the choice of proteins, vegetables, fruits, and fats being used. Follow the food sources mentioned earlier.

Since nutrition is 75% of reaching your fitness goals, try your best to stay the course.

Benefits of Juicing

One of the other tools I recommended for getting rid of excess weight is juicing. Juicing has proven to be a great way to increase energy while ridding the body of waste and bloat. Of course, the food items selected for juicing has to make sense.

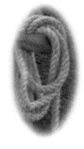

Which wouldn't include pork sausage, steak, or fried chicken. I had to go there.

I recommend you pick at least two days for total juicing. Mondays and Thursdays are the best choices. Juicing should be used for breakfast, lunch, and supper. If and when you get hungry between meals, have water and a (1) serving of fruit (apple, pear, orange, banana) or a medium mixed green salad with balsamic vinaigrette.

Not only does juicing jump start weight loss, it also leave you feeling more energized throughout your day.

My favorite juice combination of spinach (2-3 hand full), carrots (4-5 baby carrots), pineapple (3-4 squares), and 4oz of spring water.

And here's why:

> Spinach is high in in minerals such as calcium, magnesium, potassium and iron. These are important in fighting muscle fatigue and cardio-vascular health.

> Carrots are high in beta-carotene, which promotes cellular health to fight disease.

> Pineapple is known to have several benefits such as aiding digestion, fighting inflammation, increasing circulation, and adding a pleasant taste to what would have been a bitter juice combination.

Last but not least, the glue that pulls it all together, quality H2O, in the form of certified spring water.

There are several blenders or juicers on the market that work great. However, I prefer the Magic Bullet. It is affordable and easy to use. I also like that it comes with a recipe guide that showcases information on additional juicing combinations.

Give your body the nutrition needed to repair and manage your age.

...

With the combined knowledge of the right nutrition, supplementation, and exercise program, fitness goals are possible at any age!

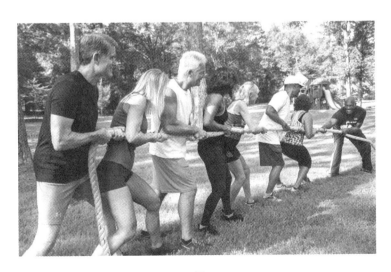

CHAPTER SIX

EXERCISE AT ANY AGE

Exercise has proven to be a must in the pursuit of long-term quality health. Yet, we struggle with making it a part of our daily routine.

Sure, exercise is uncomfortable. Laying on the sofa and watching your favorite show while sipping on a cold soda feels good.

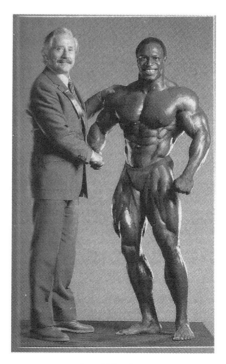

Joe Weider

There is a saying, "If you don't use it, you'll lose it." Every day that passes without exercise is a missed opportunity to add another quality day to your health.

We must draw a line in the sand, and make up our minds that we're not going down without a fight!

As I said earlier, "It's hard work being cute." It doesn't fall from the sky. You have got to go get it.

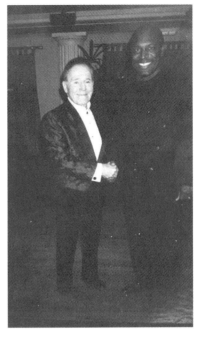

Jack LaLanne

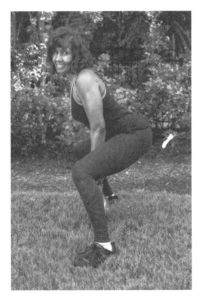

Ask Shirley, who's 70 years young, fit, and fabulous!

Your level of cuteness will be determined by your level of commitment.

The benefits of regular exercise are well worth the effort.

Feeling good, looking good, and yes, enhanced sexual performance (*percolation*) in a moment's notice, are only a few of the many benefits you gain through exercise.

69

Two of the greatest examples of the benefits of exercise were fitness icons, Joe Weider and Jack LaLanne, who both lived past 90 years old.

Also, the beautiful Ernestine Shepherd, who's still flexing into her 80's. She discovered weight training while in her mid-50s, and hasn't looked back since.

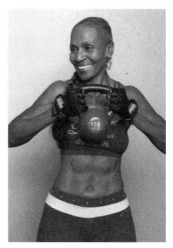

These are just a few examples of what's possible when exercise and good nutrition are a part of our daily routine.

Ernestine Shepherd

Here are some of the salient benefits of exercise:

- Produces proper blood flow throughout the body, which is important for circulation
- Helps the body burn fat more efficiently
- Helps strengthen the skeletal system by building muscle and strong bones, in the prevention of osteoporosis
- Increases stamina by strengthening lung capacity
- Creates circulation for percolation (enhanced sexual performance)

The last, but not least benefit of exercise, is that it keeps you looking young, sexy, and healthy!

There's nothing wrong with a little healthy vanity. Who wouldn't like a nice tapered waist, with buns of steel to go with it. However, exercise and nutrition on this level isn't for the faint of heart. It's hard work and consistency!

As past chairman of the President's Council on Physical Fitness and Sports, my team and I were always searching for ways to help educate people about the importance of regular exercise and proper nutrition.

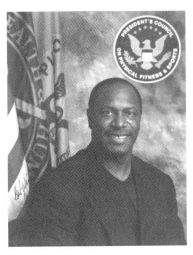

One of our top priorities was getting the word out about adult and childhood obesity. Every day, people of all ages are being diagnosed with diseases like diabetes, high blood pressure, and heart disease, with no end in sight.

President's Council

Spending too much time in front of the television, playing games on the computer, and making our top social events about food has polarized our population.

This is one of the biggest reasons behind the high cost of medical insurance. Americans are eating themselves to death. Knee and hip replacements are steadily rising, because we are carrying far too much weight.

Without a system of national accountability being offered through medical insurance providers, it will be impossible to control the cost of rising medical insurance.

Fitness incentives, perhaps rewarding people with tax breaks or lower premiums, would be a great way to get people committed. If all the insurance providers follow suite, this would make a tremendous difference. How about it folks, Lee Haney for President.

The ultimate exercise program:

Functional Training

This particular training system was created to enhance the functionality of the entire body. It challenges muscles from head to toe, while helping to increase strength, cardio condition, core muscles, flexibility, and promote continual blood flow!

After years of working with clients on every level, I've found functional training to be the answer to yielding the best results in the shortest period of time.

What is Functional Training?
Functional Training consists of a series of exercises that imitate the natural function of the body. Daily functions, such as pulling, pushing, stretching, bending, reaching, and squatting. In order to be fit, we must continuously incorporate exercises that enhance natural function and mobility. Functional Training can be used as an exercise program for adults of any age group.

Listed on the following page are four areas of concern 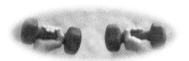 that must be trained in order to obtain true functional wellness:

- Strength Training for Stronger Muscles
- Core Training for Balance (abdominal, hips, and lower back strength)
- Flexibility Training/Stretching
- Cardiovascular Training for Stamina

Everything is connected to everything. A good example of functional wellness can be seen in the simple task of getting out of bed.

The combination of the core (abdominals, hips, and lower back) and flexibility required is a challenge itself. Plus, upper and lower body strength is necessary to sit up on the side of the bed. Then there's the strength needed to generate enough force to rise from a semi-squatting position. Lastly, cardiovascular stamina is needed to provide the endurance to complete the function.

Now that we have a clear understanding of what functional training is about, here is an explanation of the four areas to focus on.

Strength Training:
Strength training has proven to be one of the most effective ways to develop and maintain a healthy, functional body. There is something to gain from strength training, whether you're a baby boomer wanting to keep your body toned or a weekend warrior athlete, you can benefit tremendously from it!

In the sport of bodybuilding, strength training is used to develop the shape and size of muscles. With power lifting or Olympic lifting, it's used to develop explosive power, strength, and speed.

When setting up a strength training program, there are basic fundamentals that should be followed. Each muscle group has its own specific foundational strength movement.

The following is a combination of functional strength movements that make up the foundation for each major muscle group:

Biceps:
Barbell or dumbbell curls (pull)

Shoulders:
Military press using dumbbells or barbells (push)

Back:
Barbell or dumbbell rows (pull)

Chest:
Standing chest press using resistance bands or pushups military style or with knees bent to the floor for support (push)

Triceps:
Kickbacks or one arm triceps extensions using dumbbells (push)

Legs:
Dumbbell or barbell squats (push)

There are other movements that can be used; however, the ones mentioned are the bread and butter of a sound functional strength training program.

> NOTE: At the end of each exercise, push or pull characterizes the movement and its effect on the muscle group. My top choice for exercise equipment is dumbbells. I prefer free weight because they force the user to use stabilizing muscle throughout the entire body, especially in the core areas (i.e., hips, lower back, abdominals). Other equipment choices available are resistance bands, kettle bells, battle ropes, and medicine balls.

Number of Sets and Repetitions

Now that we have an understanding of what the fundamental strength movements are, let's take a look at choosing the recommended number of sets and repetitions. The goal should always be "train to stimulate, not annihilate." In other words, don't tear yourself up by putting yourself in harm's way. It's the same concept as "Drive 55 and stay alive!"

The bottom line: It's okay to challenge your fitness from time to time. However, be mindful that you're not 25.

When doing a functional training workout for the first time, the number of sets should be no more than one to two sets per exercise. The number of repetitions should range from 12-15 per set.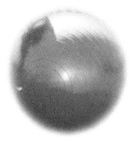

A *set* is completed when the required number of repetitions has been performed (1 set x 12 repetitions). Afterward, you will proceed to the next set.

As for rest between sets, it depends largely upon the individual. For someone who has already developed a level of endurance, they may need no more than 35-40 seconds between sets. On the other hand, someone just getting started may need 40-60 seconds of rest between sets. A great way to use the break between sets is stretching. Follow the instructions shown in the section on stretching.

Core Training:

Having a strong core is everything when it comes to being in functional shape. The core consists of the muscles located in the abdominal, lower back, and hips. These particular muscles and cardio-vascular exercises together are called secondary exercises. In no way am I downplaying their role in achieving optimum fitness. Without core strength, functional health isn't possible, no matter how physically good you look.

When muscles in these areas are properly trained, you can handle your business; however, when they're not, you're an accident waiting to happen, which nearly always show up in the form of lower back problems or hip injuries.

The core is involved in every functional movement we make, whether it's reaching for a cup, bending to pick something up, vacuuming the floor, pushing the lawn mower, pulling a branch, or doing the twist on the dance floor. It all has to do with the core, and how it connects to the total picture of true functional health.

There are several exercises to strengthen the core muscles. Since I'm a meat and (sweet) potato kind of guy, I appreciate exercises that imitate the natural function of the body's mechanics.

My first choices for safety are standing leg raises, seated leg raises, crunches, lower back extensions, and bird dogs after a level of core strength is developed.

If you are currently experiencing lower back pain, check with your doctor before trying any of these exercises, or better yet, contact the International Chiropractors Association for a healthcare provider in your area. To learn more, visit www.chiropractic.org.

A good exercise routine keeps your core strong. Start with the abs first.

I recommend lower back/core training at the end of every workout. See core training instructions shown on the Fit at Any Age link provided at www.leehaney.com.

Stretching:

Stretching is important for prevent injuries. Let's rephrase that to say "correct stretching." I use the term correct stretching because I had an associate of mine injure himself by over stretching while his muscles were still cold.

FIT AT ANY AGE

There's a methodical and proper way of stretching. When observing the natural habits of cats and dogs, one of the first things they do after waking from a nap is stretch—and they didn't read a book on the importance of stretching. Apparently, they know something we don't.

Stretching is one of the main ingredients needed to keep our bodies functional and healthy. There are basically two simple ways to incorporate proper stretching. One is by first warming the body up by doing some form of aerobic activity, such as three to five minutes of stepping in place, walking, or using the treadmill, exercise bike, or the elliptical. Afterward, slowly begin to stretch the muscles.

Another way is to stretch the muscles between every other set of strength, core, or cardiovascular (exercises). Keep in mind stretching must be done cautiously. There are many different ways to stretch the muscles. Keep it simple.

Cardiovascular Training:
Cardiovascular conditioning is one of the most important areas of functional wellness. This provides the ability to supply the body with the adequate amount of oxygen.

I've always taken the position, "It's better to have, and not need, than to need, and not have." Also keep in mind, emergencies will not wait until you catch your breath before reacting.

There are several cardio exercises that can be incorporated into a functional training program. For beginners, start with basic, non-impact cardio exercise, such as walking, using the treadmill, or using the elliptical.

A brisk 30-minute walk is a great start. The main thing is to get the blood flowing and the heart pumping.

For those who already possess a decent level of stamina with no injuries, I recommend jogging in place, jumping jacks, step-ups, high steps, back pedaling, side shuffles, skips hop, and vertical jumps.

These types of exercises not only increase cardiovascular condition, but they also help to strengthen bone density. Decide which movements best serve your goals while not putting yourself in harm's way.

Remember, "Stimulate, not Annihilate!" I repeat, the main thing is to get the blood flowing and the heart pumping.

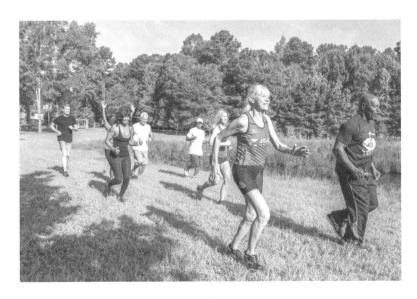

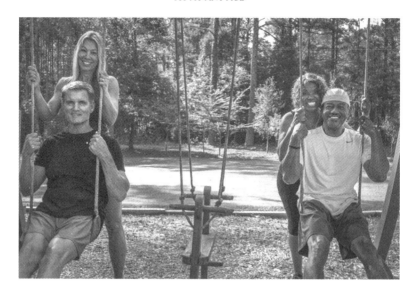

For the guys, cardiovascular training is the cheapest form of E.D. treatment in the world. "If you circulate, you percolate!"

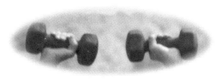

CHAPTER SEVEN

FUNCTIONAL TRAINING WORKOUT

Before getting started, be sure you have gotten the approval from your physician, and invited him or her to join you.

NOTE: The following program was created to combine the exercise tools mentioned previously. The movements used will be paired in a push/pull/core/cardio sequence.

Warm Up:
I recommend 5-10 minutes of low impact movements used to warm up prior to doing resistance exercises.

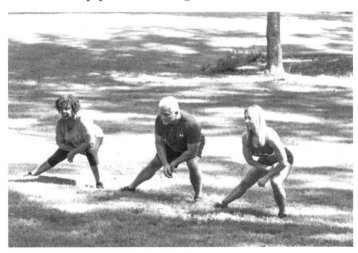

Stretching

Stretches:

With the legs spread a little more than shoulder width apart and lean to the right for a count of 6 (-1000 seconds count); then repeat the count to the left, while still in the standing position. Lower the glutes, parallel to the knees for groin stretches, for the repeated count of 6 (-1000 seconds). From the squat position, slowly lean forward, lowering the upper body with the arms extended, reaching outward toward the floor with the hamstrings. Stretch to the point of being slightly uncomfortable.

Torso side twist:

With both feet planted firmly, twist the upper body to the right and left while gently turning the feet. With each turn of the torso, complete 8-10 controlled twists to each side.

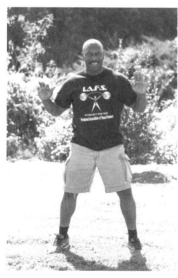 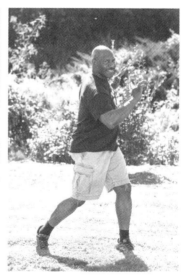

Torso Twist: Start   Finish

Lateral arm rotations forward:
Raise both arms out to the side while extended. Slowly rotate in a circular motion, clockwise, for a count of 10. Then counter-clockwise, to repeat the rotation, same as before.

Neck rotations:
While standing, gently rotate the neck clockwise for a count of 8-10, then counter-clockwise, to repeat the same count. The amount of time spent stretching may vary. I advise doing at least two sets of each movement with a 5 (-1000) count. Hold between each repetition.

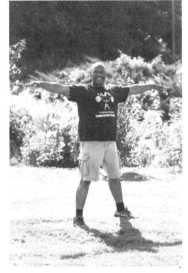

Arm Rotations: Start/Finish

Let's now move to the resistance exercises.

Biceps curl:
Barbell or dumbbell curls (pull) 1-2 sets x 15 reps

From the standing position, having dumbbells in each hand at the side of the hip area, curl the dumbbells upward towards the shoulders while flexing the biceps at the top of the movement. Then, lower them back to the start position, repeating the movement until the total number of repetitions are completed.

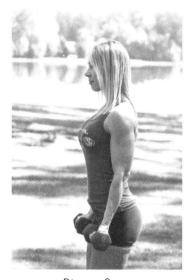
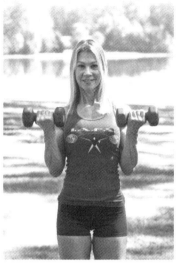

Bicep: Start   Finish

Shoulders:
Dumbbells military press (push) 1-2 sets x 15 reps

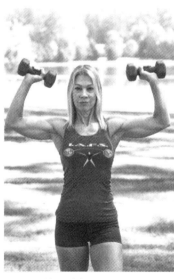
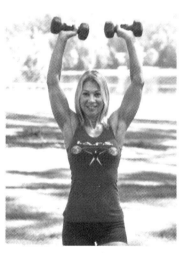

Shoulders: Start   Finish

From the standing position, raise both dumbbells parallel to the shoulders, then proceed pressing both of them over the head to complete the movement, bringing them back to the starting position.

Repeat the movement until the required number of repetitions are completed.

Core:
Standing leg raise x 15-20 reps

From the standing position with the legs shoulder width apart, raise the leg up and slightly across the body, with the knee raised, while flexing the abdominal muscles to complete the first rep to the right side (opposite side of the body).

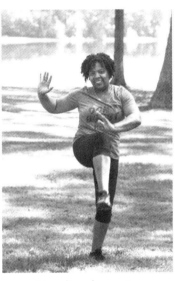

Then, repeat the exact movement to the opposite (left side) of the body to complete the total rep count of one-one, two-two, three-

Standing leg raise

three, etc. Repeat the movement until the total number of repetitions are completed.

Cardio:
Stepping in place (45-60 sec.)

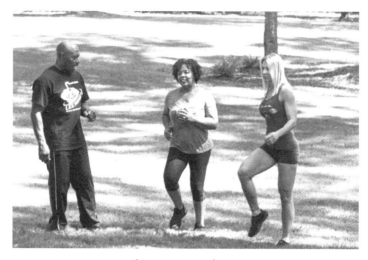

Stepping in place

Stepping in place is as simple as marching in the same spot, or if there's room, a swift walk around a fixed perimeter is fine. Be sure to wear good quality shoes.

Stretching (hamstring, groin, and glutes):
With the legs spread a little more than shoulder width apart, lean to the right for a count of 6 (-1000). Count,

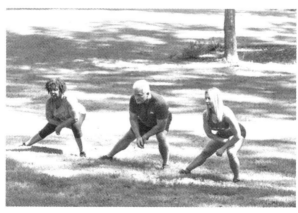

Stretching

then repeat the count to the left, while still in the standing position. Lower the glutes parallel to the knees for groin stretches, for the repeated count of 6 (-1000).

From the squat position, slowly lean forward, lowering the upper body, with the arms extended, reaching outward towards the floor with the hamstrings. Stretch to the point of being slightly uncomfortable.

Back:
   Dumbbell rows (pull) 1-2 sets x 15 reps

In a standing 45-degree position, holding two dumbbells with the back slightly arched with the shoulders back, raise the dumbbells upward simultaneously on the both sides, squeezing the back muscles in the center. Then, lower the dumbbells back to the starting position to complete the movement.

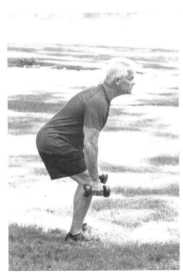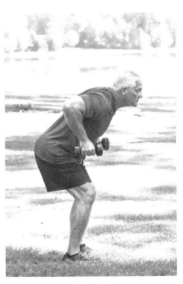

 Dumbbell: Start   Finish

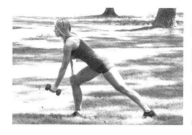 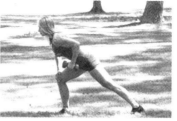

One arm dumbbell: Start   Finish

One arm dumbbell rows is an alternative to the two hand rows. They are performed by positioning the body in a 45-degree angle with the back bent and leg extended on the side to which the dumbbell is placed in hand. The opposite leg and elbow should act to give balance while in the rowing position. With the arm extended, pull the dumbbell upward to the side while squeezing the upper and lower back muscles.

Repeat the movement until the recommended repetitions are completed on both sides of the back.

Chest:
> Standing resistance band or pushups (push) 1-2 sets x 12-15 reps

Place the resistant band around the upper back. With the hands gripping the handles with the inner palms, press the band outward in a pushing motion, working the chest muscles. Then, slowly lower the band back to the starting position to complete the movement.

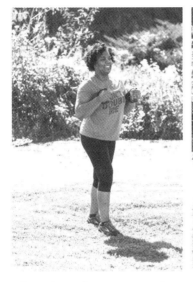

Standing chest press with
bands: Start

Finish

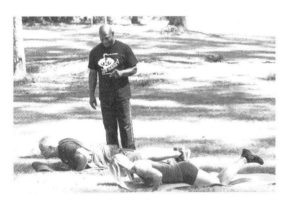

Pushups: Start

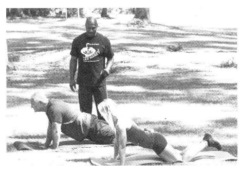

Finish

Core:
Crunches or standing leg raise x 15-20 reps

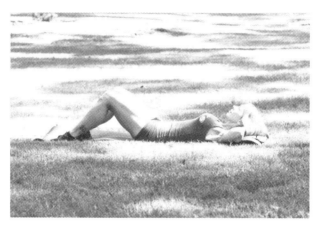

Crunches: Start

While lying on the back with the knees bent, feet flat on the floor, hands to the side of each ear, curl upward towards the ceiling, flexing the abdominal muscles, then return to the starting position until the recommended number of repetitions are complete.

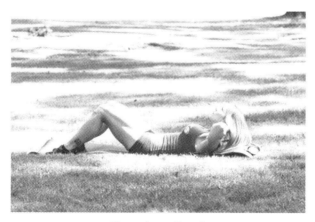

Crunches: Finish

Triceps:
Kickbacks or one-arm triceps extensions using dumbbells (push) 1-2 sets x 15 reps

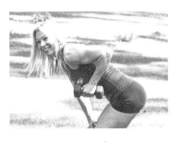 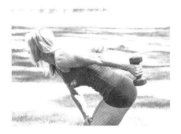

Triceps: Start   Finish

In a 45-degree standing angle, with the back slightly arched, hold the dumbbell with the right hand, elbow locked to the right side. Slowly extend the elbow back towards the rear, flexing the back of the arm (triceps), then bring it back to the starting position to complete the recommended number of repetitions, then proceed to the opposite arm.

Legs:
Dumbbell squats (push) 1-2 sets x 15 reps

From the standing position while holding dumbbells in both hands, head straight ahead, feet flat on the floor with heals planted, lower the body into a squatting position while keeping the gluts over the heels.

Squat until reaching the sitting position (parallel), then, without hesitation, press upward, back into the starting position to complete the movement.

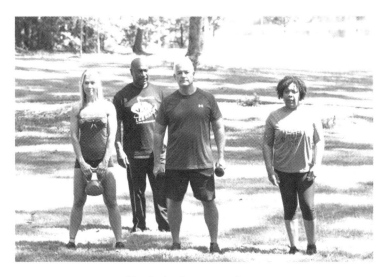

Kettle bell squats: Start

Repeat until the recommended number of repetitions are complete.

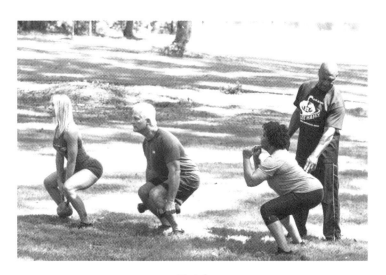

Finish

Stretching:

Lunge to left/right/middle 6 (-1000 second) count intervals

Core:

Standing leg raise x 15-20 reps

From the standing position with the legs shoulder width apart, raise the leg up and slightly across the body, with the knee raised, while flexing the abdominal muscles to complete the first rep to the right side (opposite side of the body). Then, repeat the exact movement to the opposite (left side) of the body to complete the total rep count of one-one, two-two, three-three, etc. Repeat the movement until the total number of repetitions are completed.

Cardio:

Battle rope (45-60 sec.)

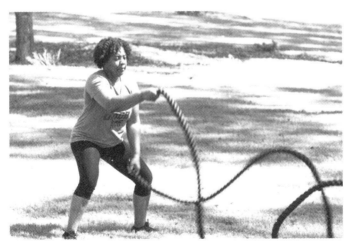

Battle ropes

Battle rope training is excellent as a cardio choice while giving the knees and hips a rest from stress brought on by over use. I especially recommend it to people suffering from knee or hip discomfort.

Simply hold the ropes while alternating it up and down or simultaneously raising the rope up and down in a rhythm like sequence in a similar way for a 45 to 60 second count.

To add to the functional training workout, I recommend back extensions and or bird dogs. Both are excellent exercises design to strengthen stabilization muscles in the lower back/core area.

Back extensions:
These are done while lying flat on the stomach, with both hands and legs extended outward. While extended, raise both hands and legs 2 inches off

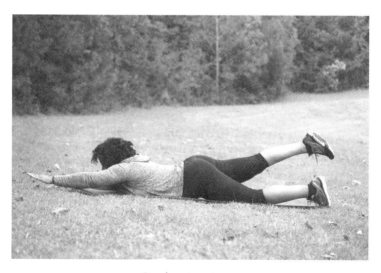

Back extensions

the floor, holding for a count of 6 (-1000). Example: (1-1000, 2-1000, 3-1000, etc.). Proceed to do two to three sets.

Bird Dogs:

While on all fours in a doggy style position, raise right hand and extend the opposite left leg for a count of 5-6 (-1000) (same as previous exercise) for a total of two or three sets.

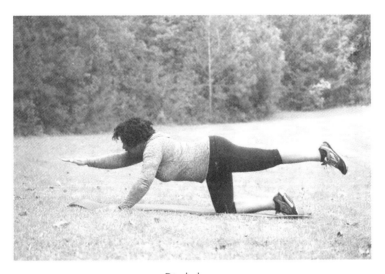

Bird dogs

· · ·

This completes the functional training exercise sequence.

See the functional training Fit At Any Age link for visual instructions explaining proper form using the listed exercises at www.leehaney.com.

> NOTE: Be sure to have cool or room temperature water available during the workout to sip as needed. Do not guzzle. If you experience dizziness while exercising, stop and cool down. Should the dizziness persist, seek help or call 911.

When it comes to training programs, this is the all-time greatest. It is straight to the point, and generally takes less than 30 minutes to complete.

> NOTE: All of the listed exercises are performed in a standing position, which helps to strengthen the core, and stabilizes muscles. This, in fact, should be the normal way of exercising.

However, if you are physically challenged, functional training is still possible in a sitting position. A few years ago, I had a female client who was confined to using a walker due to weight issues. After four months of performing function training exercises and incorporating aquatics, she dropped 40 lbs.

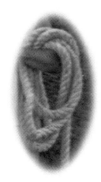

The end results were that she no longer needed the walker, regained her overall health, and discontinued some of the meds she was on.

Functional Training is the new face of fitness as it should be. It is exercise that

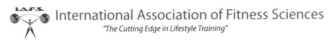

International Association of Fitness Sciences
"The Cutting Edge in Lifestyle Training"

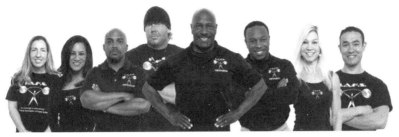

helps maintain functionality at any age, while increasing overall functionality.

I am so convinced about the benefits of Functional training I created what is now The International Association of Fitness Science (I.A.F.S.).

The I.A.F.S. offers a Functional Training/Basic Nutrition certification for those who desire to impact the lives of people and communities. The I.A.F.S. has given its trainers the tools needed to teach functional training exercise all over the U.S.

The Functional Training/Basic Nutrition certification is also available packaged as the Minister of Fitness certification, which is being offered to community churches and other places of worship.

For more information concerning our personal training course, visit www.iafscertification.com.

Dealing with Injury:

The best thing to do in case of an injury is don't have one. Most people get injured from using too much weight, or not properly warming up.

One of the most important things to remember when it comes to exercise is moderation. "Stimulate, not annihilate!" You don't have to tear yourself up to get great fitness results. And by all means, don't allow a wet-behind-the-ears trainer cause you to get injured. Warning: If it doesn't feel right, it isn't right. Don't do it. Let the trainer know, unapologetically.

When and if an injury occurs, treat the inflamed area with an ice or cold gel pack. This will help ease swelling and reduce pain in the first 24 hours. If the pain continues, contact your physician.

Motivation:

Staying healthy has to do with having a positive mindset. I often use the phrase "Get your mind right" when my wife, Shirley, and I prepare to lead our Grown Folks Boot Camp.

People often struggle with finding a reason to stay on task when it comes to taking care of their health. In order to stick and stay, we have to find our personal "Why!"

For some, it might be living longer, feeling better, or fulfilling your bucket list.

For others, it might be the personal vanity of looking good. Staying cute is not easy. It takes intentional time spent exercising and eating the right food.

For anyone who is a business owner, it's extremely important to be and stay healthy. After all, you are your own personal economic enterprise. If you're sick due to health issues, productivity slows or halts.

As we all know, bad health can eat away at savings in a matter of weeks, and in most cases, days. All the more reason to stay on task with your why—which should be your must.

Whatever your "Why" is, draw strength from it and own it every time you need that extra push to keep going. For me, I like looking and feeling fit—as do the Boomers gracing the cover.

Dealing with Stress:

Being able to deal with the ups and downs of life can take its toll. It's amazing how a negative comment or an unexpected occurrence can alter how we feel in a matter of seconds, raising our blood pressure, causing us to panic, or stealing our joy. I've been there many times, and so have we all.

In my 50-plus years, I've learned to deal with these never-ending situations in several ways.

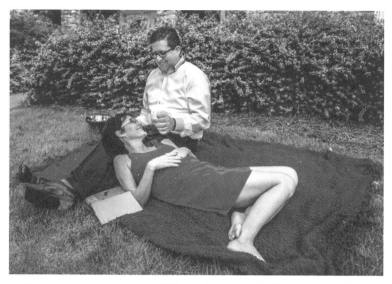

Cancer survivor Renee (53) and husband, David (51) Casey

It can be anything from walking in the park to hear birds sing, to watching children play, listening to soothing music, or hearing a motivational message.

My wife and I love breaking away for lunch in the park, or running off to a movie. We all have a choice in finding what works best for us individually.

As a follower of Jesus Christ, I've learned to lay every concern at His feet.

No matter what I'm facing, there's a place of peace that I find when I give my concerns to Him in prayer and stand on his word.

One of my favorite passages of scripture is Philippians 4:4-8, which talks about the power of surrendering worries to God in prayer when facing various challenges.

Then there's I Peter 5:7-9, which tells us to cast all of our cares up Him (Jesus), for He cares for us and our every situation.

Besides, most of the things we worry about are things that haven't actually happened. They find room in our mind, and reap havoc on our bodies.

Another vital tool for managing stress is being able to take time out for vacations.

Enjoying time with family and friends, laughing, and sharing precious memories together is key. In my international travels, I've noticed how European citizens schedule time to relax and fellowship with friends and family on a regular basis.

One of my favorite places to visit is Italy. The food, the culture, and the joys of living are so beautiful. Lunch in the town squares is filled with people laughing, drinking coffee, and sharing stories. In one of my past visits, I gained 10 lbs. in two weeks. Of course, it was healthy weight.

I've heard it said, "In order to live, you got to live!"

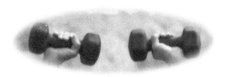

CONCLUSION

Now that we've learned how to eat, what to eat, the benefits of exercises needed to enhance functionality, and the best way to implement them, we are on our way to living out the next chapter in our journey with just as much enthusiasm as we did in the first half! Of course, we're not going to live forever. However, that doesn't mean we shouldn't think, act, talk, and live like it!

I want it said of me, "I saw Lee Haney yesterday at the gym. He looked great, and is still fully functional at the age of 95. Man, he got the best of quality and quantity."

Now, that's the way to go.

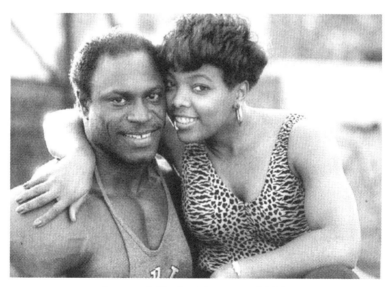

Lee and Shirley Haney in 1983

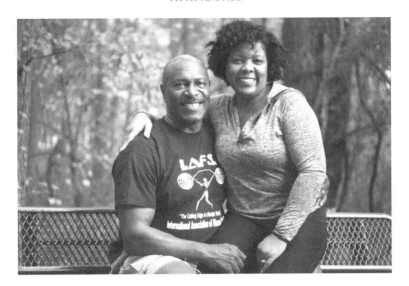

Lee and Shirley Haney today

Let's all make sure our "last set is our best set" by being fit at any age!

"Beloved, I pray that you may prosper in all things and be in health, just as your soul prospers."
– 3 John 2 (NKJV)

FIT AT ANY AGE
GOALS

What are your goals at your age? From the foods you eat to the exercises you want to do to the lifestyle you want to live, list some of those goals here:

3-Month Goals:

_____

_____

_____

_____

_____

_____

6-Month Goals:

_____

_____

_____

_____

_____

12-Month Goals:

_____

_____

_____

_____

_____

Let's get practical. What steps are you taking that will help you reach your goals? List those steps here:

_____

_____

_____

_____

_____

_____

_____

_____

_____

_____

_____

_____

_____

_____

_____

_____

_____

_____

_____

_____

_____

_____

_____

_____

FIT AT ANY AGE
LETTER OF COMMITMENT

I _____ commit
to the exercise and nutrition goals I have listed on the
previous page.

I will commit to follow the knowledge shared within the
pages of *Fit at Any Age* and learn additional fitness
information by becoming a member of Lee Haney's fitness
community available at www.leehaney.com

Date: _____

Signature: _____

FIT AT ANY AGE
CHECKLIST FOR LIFE

This is the "Icing on the Cake List" for you:

1. Start your day with a morning prayer or meditation of your choosing.

2. Prepare your meals for the day to include breakfast, snacks, lunch, and dinner.

3. Have your exercise time set in stone, not allowing any deviation in the allotted time scheduled.

4. Be sure to stay hydrated with quality water. It's easy to forget to drink the recommended 8-10 glasses of water per day.

5. Set aside time for a daily power nap to reboot your body and mind. After lunch is always a great time. Besides, the body naturally craves it.

6. Keep your heart in tune by whispering a prayer as you make your way through the day. It will keep your mind in a place of peace.

7. Finish your day with thanksgiving, even in the most challenging times. We can always find something to be thankful about no matter the circumstances.

8. I recommend keeping a daily log of your activities, meals, prayers and people you prayed for, and things you are most thankful for.

To add to your fitness experience,
I encourage you to visit www.leehaney.com
to join the community where we post
Fit At Any Age workout videos and
other fitness resources.

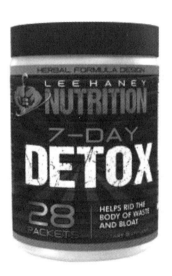

7 Day Systemic Cleansing and Detox: Combines a
mixture of herbs and other nutrients that help cleanse the
internal organs and getting rid of waste and bloat
throughout the body

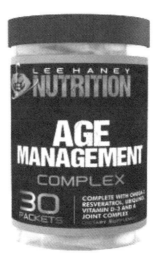

Age Management Complex: Combines a combination of nutrients to help manage age in adults of all ages.

- Vitamin D-3: Promotes bone health along with other wellness benefits. Highly recommended for preventing bone loss.
- Omega-3: Formulated to promote cardio-vascular wellness by helping the body establish healthy cholesterol levels.
- Glucosamine Sulfate, MSM, Chondroitin Sulfate for added joint health and support
- Ubiquinol: Supports cardio-vascular health while enhancing endurance and recovery. Ubiquinol is also being used to help lower blood pressure.
- Resveratrol: Known for its age management abilities. It's by far one of the most sought-after nutrients among health and fitness enthusiasts in the know.

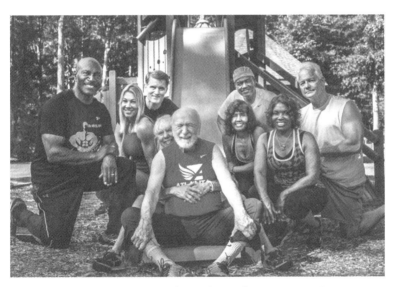

You too can get fit and stay fit at any age!

Join the
FIT AT ANY AGE
community!

For more information on Lee Haney, Lee Haney
Nutrition Products, or to have Lee Haney speak at
events, fitness workshops, and corporate wellness
functions, visit:

www.LeeHaney.com